Essential Oil Healing Secrets

ADISH Books

Copyright © 2013 ADISH Books

ISBN-13: 978-1495435317

ISBN-10: 1495435318

Disclaimer

The information specified throughout this book is provided for general information only, and should not be treated as a substitute for the medical advice of your own doctor, psychiatrist, medical counselor or any other health care professional. Nothing contained on this book is intended to be for medical diagnosis or treatment. By following the instructions contained herein, the reader willingly assumes all risks in connection with such instructions. If you think you have a medical emergency, call your doctor immediately.

WHAT IS AROMATHERAPY?..5

DIFFERENCE BETWEEN ESSENTIAL OILS AND CARRIER OILS 8

WHY USE PURE ESSENTIAL OILS?..10

HOW TO USE ESSENTIAL OILS 13

PRECAUTIONS ... WHAT CAN'T YOU DO..20

RECOGNIZING AUTHENTICITY, DIVERSITY, FRAGRANCE..................................23

HOW TO STORE YOUR ESSENTIAL OILS 25

WHERE TO PURCHASE?..27

ESSENTIAL OIL - HEALING RECIPES 31

COMMON ESSENTIAL OILS FOR HEALING 34
TREATMENT FOR SKIN, HAIR AND BODY PROBLEMS 36
Allergic Reactions Treatment 36
Broken Capillaries Treatment 38
Bruises Treatment..40
Treatment of Skin Injuries 41
Prevention of UV Damage..42
Caring for Ageing Skin..43
Treatment of Eczema 44
Treatment of Psoriasis 46
Blackheads 47
Treatment of Acne 49
Treatment of Oily skin..51
Treatment of Body Odor 52
Treatment for Brittle Nails 53
Treatment for Dandruff..54
Scar and Stretch Mark Reduction 55
Treatment of Wrinkles 56
Dry Skin 58
Treatment of Arthritis 60
Treatment of Abdominal Cramping or Pain..61
Treatment of Acid Reflux..62
Treatment Cold and Flu..63

Treatment of Depression and Sadness *64*

Treatment of Fever *65*

Treatment of Inflammation *66*

Stress Relief *67*

Treatment of Fatigue *68*

Treatment of Anxiety *69*

Headaches *70*

Treatment of Insect Bites and Stings *71*

Treatment of Back Problems *72*

Treatment of Hormonal Transitions (Menopause and PMS) *73*

Pain Relief *74*

Respiratory Conditions *75*

What Is Aromatherapy?

Aromatherapy is the use of distilled oils from plants called "essential oils" for healing purposes. The aromas of these oils can be spread in an area via a diffuser, inhaled directly, or applied topically on the skin.

Evidence for the use of herb oils as treatment dates back thousands of years to ancient Egypt, Greece, Persia and China. The ancient Egyptians were the first culture to use plant fragrances as perfume and put great stock in scent as an indicator of health. They were also the first to distill oils from plants and wood, and regularly used oils and lotions as protection from hot and dry conditions. Hippocrates, the "father of modern medicine", collected experimental data on the healing properties of hundreds of plants and herbs in his medical encyclopedia, the Hippocratic Corpus. Dioscorides did the same with his De Materia Medica, five volumes devoted almost entirely to the healing properties of herbs.

The use of aromatics and herbal remedies was also common in Persia and herbal healing properties were similarly documented by the physicians Al-Razi and Ibn Sina. The Crusades would import some of this knowledge and practice to Europe via returning soldiers. And herbal extracts and the use of aromas to calm patients and promote overall well-being has been a cornerstone of traditional Chinese medicine for thousands of years. The modern conception of "aromatherapy" begins with French scientist René-Maurice Gattefossé, however, and his publications on the therapeutic value of oils in the early twentieth century (in which he coins the term.)

The basic theory behind aromatherapy's function is that the part of the brain that controls memories and emotions is stimulated in different ways by different scents. When this stimulation occurs, the body releases chemicals and hormones that can have beneficial effects - relaxing, calming, energizing, clarifying and sharpening thought, and even promoting physical healing. The overall effect is determined by the oil or blend of oils used and the method of application. Aromatherapy also covers the topical application of these oils which can interact with the skin and be metabolized by the body.

Products marketed as being for "aromatherapy" sometimes use synthetic chemicals that do nothing but create a particular fragrance. While they can be pleasant, these are more like a perfume or air freshener than a method of health treatment. The particular compounds in plant oil concentrates are what give the essential oils their healing properties. A synthetic oil or fragrance cannot provide the same beneficial stimulation that distilled oils from plants and herbs do.

Difference between Essential Oils and Carrier Oils

An essential oil refers to any concentrated oil extracted from a plant or herb. A carrier oil, on the other hand, is a base used to dilute the strength of an essential oil. They also do not evaporate, and are thus used to preserve the potency of essential oils as they are applied.

Carrier oils generally do not have a fragrance of their own, but they do have their own therapeutic properties in combination with essential oils.

Many of the most commonly used carrier oils are those that are also favored in cooking. Cold-pressed olive, sesame, sunflower and canola oil are all commonly used as carrier oils. Oils from nuts - almond, macadamia, walnut, pecan and peanut - can also be used as carrier oils, though potentially deadly nut allergies must be considered.

Other potential carrier oils include jojoba,

emu, castor, evening primrose and grape seed oils. While every carrier oil has its own unique properties, in general they are good sources of Omega 3 fatty acids, antioxidants and nutrients.

Why use Pure Essential Oils?

When it comes to essential oils, purity is the main determinant of quality. Some oils marketed as "essential" are actually cut with synthetic chemicals that are cheaper to manufacture than genuine oil extract. Other considerations are how long (and in what type of containers) the oil has been stored, and whether the plants the extract was taken from were grown in optimal conditions or treated with pesticides.

There are few governmental organizations worldwide that are testing and regulating essential oils. The United States FDA will test essential oils if they are marketed as an ingestible product or as an aid in treating a medical condition, but very few are marketed that way. France's AFNOR is a bit more rigorous about testing the contents of oils, including any that are imported into Europe.

The best way to find pure essential oils is to examine the reputation of the company providing them. Signs to look for in a company is a clear statement of 100% purity on the packaging, the precise Latin name of the plant species provided, and companies that are open about their growing process and extraction technique (i.e., they've let people in to see it and document it before, such as for a news or magazine story.) If an oil is very inexpensive compared to other similar oils, it's a big red flag. The use of the term "grade" is also something to investigate with caution as there are no regulatory bodies that provide official grades for essential oil.

The country of origin is also very important. Is the plant in question actually grown in the country that the oil is manufactured in, or at least in a neighboring country? With their stronger regulations, countries in the European Union are also generally a safer bet.

An aromatherapy expert can tell you which countries are best to look to for the particular herbal extracts you need.

How to Use Essential Oils

There are a number of methods for using essential oils:

Topical Application

Topical application is simply the direct application of oils to the skin. This is where the carrier oils mention before come into play, as applying undiluted oil directly to the skin is generally not beneficial and may produce adverse results.

Aromatherapy recipes sometimes do call for direct application of undiluted oil, however. When they do they will use the word "neat" (like a glass of scotch straight up without ice or water.) Topical oils will more often need to be diluted with a carrier oil. The two common exceptions to this rule are lavender and tea tree oil, which are safe to apply directly to skin and beneficial in healing minor wounds.

An aromatherapist should be consulted before any new topical application, but generally carrier oil will be applied in a much greater ratio to the essential oil being applied. Application is generally by gentle rubbing or by compress.

Inhalation

The simplest method of inhalation is to apply the oil directly to a cotton ball and sniff it. This method can also be used for a light ambient application, by applying a stronger dose of oil to the cotton ball (or to multiple cotton balls) and leaving them around the area you are relaxing in.

For a stronger inhalation method you can apply drops of the oil to a steaming bowl of water. With a towel over your head and the bowl, keep your eyes closed and take a deep breath then uncover. Since this is a very potent method, it's best to consult an aromatherapy expert about dosage before using it. If in doubt, use only one drop of oil. More than two will probably not be necessary.

Diffusion

It's important not to directly heat an essential oil if it is being used for treatment, as direct flame can burn the oil and break down important compounds. If you want an automated and ambient use of your essential oils, you'll want to invest in a diffuser.

Diffusers emit a continual stream of vaporized essential oil into the air. They often come with timers. There are four basic types of diffuser on the market: evaporative, heat, humidifying and nebulizing. Nebulizers work on the same principles as a perfume atomizer and are generally seen as the optimal type for health treatments, as they put a higher concentration of oil into the air. However, they are also generally the noisiest and require larger amounts of oil to operate as they are designed to permeate entire rooms. Heat diffusers gently evaporate the oil at a low temperature, and run with no sound at all.

Evaporative diffusers are also generally very quiet, using a small fan to very quickly evaporate the oil and send it into the air. Their downside is that this method disperses the compounds in the oil more unevenly. Humidifying diffusers create a mist of pure essential oil, but require some form of air flow in the room to actually disperse.

Ingestion

Though some essential oils are safe to ingest in very small doses of 1 to 2 drops, there are enough exceptions that ingestion of any oil is not recommended without first consulting an experienced aromatherapist.

While it may seem instinctive as to which oils are safe to ingest, instincts can be misleading. For example, you might think wintergreen is safe, as it is used as a flavoring and in chewing gum. However, the amounts used in gum and foods are only tiny fractions of one drop. Ingesting one whole drop of wintergreen oil is enough to make you ill. Similarly, several drops of peppermint oil is enough to be toxic and to give you headaches and accelerated heartbeat. The doses present in one or two drops of oil are very often much higher than those commonly used in food products.

If oil is to be ingested, it is usually heavily diluted by being added to a glass of water or a hot tea. Chamomile and lemon oils are commonly used to make tea, and it is generally safe to add one or two drops of them to a beverage so long as you do not have allergies to them.

When it comes to ingestion, better safe than sorry. If there's any doubt at all in your mind, consult a professional aromatherapist first.

Precautions ... What Can't You Do

It has been said before, but it bears repeating: **essential oils should not be ingested except** under the advice and direction of a qualified and experienced aromatherapist.

Undiluted oils should not be applied to skin except under care of an aromatherapist. Applying oils directly to skin can lead to a permanent form of contact dermatitis called "sensitization" which will cause the skin to break out in a rash whenever it comes in contact with the oil or its source plant. More severe cases of sensitization have led to breathing problems and shock.

Oils such as tea tree may be recommended for direct application to wounds and burns. **Before applying a "patch test" should be done** by applying one drop to an inconspicuous area of the body and covering with a bandage for at least a day. Do not further apply the oil if itching or redness occurs.

If an essential oil is accidentally dripped onto skin, dilute with vegetable oil or milk before washing the area with soap and water.

Children under seven years old should not use the steam method of inhalation as it can damage their eyes. For children older than seven, use some sort of goggles that enclose the eyes (such as swimming goggles) as a precaution. Adults should close their eyes as a precaution when directly inhaling essential oils.

If essential oils make contact with the eyes, do not use water to flush them. Instead use milk or vegetable oil and seek medical attention if a burning or stinging sensation persists after flushing.

Certain oils (such as the citrus-based ones) can cause skin pigmentation if exposed to sunlight.

Some essential oils are considered hazardous

waste by the Environmental Protection Agency, as they can do serious damage if they enter waterways. A reputable vendor of oils should be able to supply a Material Safety Data Sheet for any oil that requires special disposal, and you can also find these online.

An allergy panel is not a bad idea before experimenting with essential oils for the first time.

Essential oils are highly flammable; keep them away from direct heat sources.

It is advisable to seek specialists opinion before using essential oil. As these oils are very potent so **pregnant women, infants and persons suffering from critical medical conditions should not use these methods at all.**

Recognizing Authenticity, Diversity, Fragrance

The production of essential oils is expensive as it takes pounds of plant material to produce only a relatively small amount of oil. Thus some companies have found it more profitable to dilute essential oil with synthetics that smell similar, or sometimes to concoct entirely synthetic formulas with a similar smell to that of an essential oil.

The smell of an essential oil can help you to tell the difference between something that is entirely synthetic and something that contains true essential oil. You will usually instinctively recognize a compound that is entirely synthetic as being "off" or not natural when you smell it. However, things get trickier when a product is a mix of synthetic components and some amount of actual essential oil. You may not be able to tell the difference simply by smelling them.

The simplest way to tell if oil is a pure

essential oil is if it has an ingredients list, or at least says "100% essential oil" or something of that nature on the label. As mentioned before, however, regulation of essential oils is rather lax and ingredients lists are usually not mandatory. The next best method is to research the reputation of the company you are buying from. Do they have an online presence? Are they transparent about their production process? Have they been featured in any articles? Do they have reviews from other customers?

While price alone isn't a failsafe indication of purity, the "good stuff" is always going to be among the more pricey options simply because it is expensive to make. You can weed out the choices that are suspiciously much cheaper than the other options. Another sign of a quality operation to look for is the storage and shipping of oils in dark-colored glass jars and bottles. Oil stored in clear glass will lose potency much more rapidly, and some oils can eat through plastic containers over time.

How to Store Your Essential Oils

Essential oils should always be stored in a tinted or dark-colored glass container. UV light causes the oils to oxidize and break down much faster. For this reason, oils should also be stored in a cool dark place where the temperature does not fluctuate very much, as heating and cooling also speeds up the oxidation process. The refrigerator is an ideal place for long-term storage, provided it isn't kept too cold (no colder than 5 degrees Celsius.) Some oils may become solid when stored in the refrigerator; this is nothing to worry about and does not cause damage, they simply need to be "thawed" by being left out on a counter for a bit prior to use.

It's also important to keep the caps tightly screwed on your essential oil bottles, as they will evaporate if exposed to the air. Carrier oils are less prone to evaporation, but you'll want to keep them covered anyway to avoid contamination. Most carrier oils contain unsaturated fatty acids and will require refrigeration so as not to go rancid. If you want a carrier oil that can be stored safely for years at room temperature, try coconut oil (which is also great for your skin!)

Different types of oils also have different shelf lives. In general, the citrus-based oils will break down the most quickly, beginning to lose their beneficial properties within a year even if stored under optimal conditions.

Oils should also not be stored in bottles that contain a rubber eyedropper. The oil will eventually break down the rubber in the dropper, which then mixes with the oil and contaminates it.

Where to Purchase?

Essential oils can be purchased both online and in "brick and mortar" stores.

If you are looking to shop locally, essential oils can often be found at health food stores, more "upscale" grocery stores, food co-ops, and herb shops. If you live in a heavily populated area, one helpful way to quickly identify shops that sell essential oils is to search for the term on yelp.com. This tends to work a lot better in cities, however; more rural and low in population an area is, the less Yelpers there tend to be. In those areas you may have to resort to the old-fashioned method of digging out the phone book and calling stores that seem likely to sell essential oils.

Some of the nationwide retail chains carry essential oils, though you will need to do your own diligence about the quality. Selection and availability may also vary by location, but many of these stores also have essential oils listed on their websites for online orders or store pickup. Retailers that carry at least a small selection of essential oils include:

- Walgreens
- Whole Foods
- Trader Joe's
- GNC
- Sprouts
- CVS Pharmacy
- Walmart
- Target
- Hobby Lobby
- Vitamin Shoppe
- Vitamin World
- Wegmans

If you're shopping online, there are many more options. There are many small specialty retailers that either produce their own oils or resell high-quality oils. Here is a partial list to begin your investigation with:

- Bramble Berry

(www.brambleberry.com/Essential-Oils-C157.aspx)

- Mountain Rose Herbs
  (www.mountainroseherbs.com/)
- Veriditas Botanicals
  (http://veriditasbotanicals.com/oils_lav.html)
- AuraCacia
  (http://www.auracacia.com/auracacia/art.html)
- Floracopeia (http://www.floracopeia.com/)
- The Oil Shop (http://www.experience-essential-oils-shop.com/)
- Timeless Apothecary
  (www.timelessessentialoils.com/)
- Simplers Botanicals
  (http://www.shopsimplers.com/)
- LorAnn Oils (www.lorannoils.com/)
- San Francisco Herb Company
  (http://www.sfherb.com/)

The larger online retailers also sometimes

carry a range of essential oils. You can find essential oils for sale at the following online retailers:

- Amazon.com (may be sold either direct from Amazon or by third-party vendors)
- Drugstore.com
- eBay.com (sold by individuals and businesses rather than by eBay themselves)
- Overstock.com
- Soap.com

Essential Oil - Healing Recipes

The concentrated extracts derived from blossoms, roots, seeds or leaves of plants are known as essential oils. These oils have their own set of active ingredients that determine the healing properties of the oil. While some essential oils heal physically, others heal emotionally. Therefore, while one essential oil may heal the swelling of your feet, another may calm you down. For example, orange essential oil has an active ingredient that will calm you down.

Using essential oils for healing is known as aromatherapy. The word aromatherapy may lead you to believe that the oils have to be inhaled. But, you can massage them on your skin too. Whether you inhale them or apply them on your skin, these oils have been found to treat stress, infections and many other problems.

It is not clearly known how essential oils heal. It is believed that the oils affect the sensory organs, such as our nose, to heal. The nose has smell reception that communicates with the brain. The parts of brain that are emotional and memory storehouses (hippocampus and amygdale) further promote treatment. The molecules of essential oils, which you inhale, stimulate the brain and affect mental, emotional and physical health.

For example, lavender; it is believed that it has sedative properties. Scientists believe that the active ingredients in lavender cause a smell that stimulates the amygdale, helping a person to sleep.

When massaged on the body, the essential oils are soothing and relaxing. They serve a dual purpose. While, on one hand, they are absorbed by skin, on the other hand, the smell stimulates the brain and promotes healing.

Massaging – Essential oils such as orange, rose, bergamot, sandalwood and many others are massaged on the body. They can be used for various purposes such as relieving headache, body or joint pains or improve moods. A few drops of the oil chosen for treatment is warmed between the palms and massaged on the body in circular motion. Skin absorbs the oils and promotes healing.

Inhaling – Essential oils are also used by means of inhaling. A few drops of oil are added along with water in a diffuser and heated gently. The aroma that spreads is inhaled and promotes healing. In certain cases, the oil is also added in a vaporizer for inhalation.

Common Essential Oils for Healing

Essential oils are extracted from plants and are very effective in treatment of various ailments – physical and medical. There are various essential oils and each of them has a different property that treats a particular or multiple conditions. Here are some commonly used essential oils for healing –

- Lavender Oil

- Carrot Seed Oil

- Chamomile Oil

- Cypress Oil

- Eucalyptus Oil

- Helichrysum Oil

- Lavender Oil

- Geranium Oil

- Marjoram Oil

- Mandarin Oil

- Myrrh Oil

- Frankincense Oil

- Peppermint Oil

- Tea tree Oil

A few drops of these oils are used in combination with carrier oils and then applied topically or inhaled for treatment. Here are a few essential oil recipes -

Treatment for skin, hair and body problems

Allergic Reactions Treatment

Basically, three essential oils are popularly used to treat allergic reactions. This can be the sneezing and itching that accompanies the change in weather or other allergies. These three oils combine to give you an effective remedy for your allergies. They are so effective that when you begin to use them, you will find them to be a substitution for the drugs that you would normally use.

Ingredients:

- Lavender Oil
- Lemon Oil
- Peppermint Oil

Directions:

Recipe 1

Mix 3 drops each of the oils to one glass of water or juice. Swish inside your mouth for about 20 seconds and then swallow.

Recipe 2

Take an empty vegetable capsule and add 5 drops of each of the oils in it. Swallow. The empty capsule will be available at your store where you get health foods.

Recipe 3

Take one drop each of the oils and add to one teaspoon of honey. Swallow.

Since these oils are for consumption, you will have to ensure that the oils are CPTG doTerra oils. If you do not find these oils that can be taken internally, then just apply a mixture of the oils on your foot soles and cover with socks.

Broken capillaries are often visible on mature skin. The following two essential oil recipes are helpful in the treatment of broken capillaries.

<u>Recipe 1</u>

Ingredients:

- Rosehip seed oil (1/2 ounce)
- Jojoba oil (1 ounce)
- Borage oil (10 drops)
- Lemon oil (3 drops)
- Cypress oil (4 drops)
- Palmarosa oil (2 drops)

Directions:

Mix the Rosehip seed and jojoba oil in a clean bowl. When they are well mixed, add the other oils. Shake well so that the oils are well mixed.

To Use:

Take a few drops of the mixture and apply on the broken capillaries twice a day.

Recipe 2

Ingredients:

- Rosehip seed oil and Hazelnut oil (1/4 ounce each)
- Borage oil (10 drops)
- Rose oil and neroli oil (3 drops each)
- Geranium oil (2 drops)

Directions:

Mix rosehip seed, hazelnut and borage oil in a clean glass bowl. When these oils are well mixed, add the remaining oils. Shake well so that they are completely mixed.

To Use:

Apply a few drops of this floral mixture to the broken capillaries once a day.

Bruises Treatment

Helichrysum Essential oil is one of the best oils used in the treatment of bruises, including sports bruises. This oil is also helpful in the release of emotional blocks and uplifts mood.

Ingredients:

- Jojoba oil (1 ounce)
- Helichrysum Oil (8 drops)

Directions:

Combine the two oils in a clean glass bowl or in a dark glass bottle.

To Use:

Apply a few drops of the oil on the bruises twice a day.

Treatment of Skin Injuries

Helichrysum essential oil is effective in the treatment of skin injuries also. It is going to be your skin's best friend. The oil has analgesic properties that reduce pain and thus, it is the right oil for treating skin injuries.

Ingredients:

- Jojoba oil (1 ounce)
- Helychrysum Oil (8 drops)
- Lavender (5 drops)

Directions:

Mix the oils in a clean glass bottle and shake well to mix the oil thoroughly.

To Use:

Apply a few drops of the oil on your skin. Helichrysum oil is effective in treating skin injuries.

Prevention of UV Damage

The essential oil derived from the Manuka tree has been traditionally used by New Zealanders to treat fever, pain and wound. In addition, it is also found to be effective in preventing UV damage and prevents ageing.

Ingredients

- Manuka Essential Oil

Directions:

Add two to three drops of Manuka essential oil to your bath.

To Use:

Take bath with the water to which Manuka essential oil has been added. Use it once a day for prevention of UV damage.

Frankincense essential oil, lavender essential oil and orange essential oil also help prevent skin from ultraviolet damage.

Caring for Ageing Skin

Neroli and carrot seed essential oils are known for their soothing, detoxing and skin rejuvenating properties. They are excellent for mature, oily, dry and sensitive skins. In addition, they work to reduce stretch marks and wrinkles.

Ingredients:

- Jojoba oil (1/2 ounce)

- Almond oil (1/2 ounce)

- Carrot seed oil (6-8 drops)

- Neroli Oil (6-8 drops)

Directions:

Jojoba and almond oils are carrier oils. Carrot seed and Neroli oils are essential oils. Mix the carrier oils in a dark colored glass bottle to mix the oils and shake them well. Add six to eight drops of each of the essential oils and shake well again.

To Use:

Apply a few drops of the serum to your skin once a day.

Lavender oil is one of the most popular oils used in the treatment of eczema and many other diseases. It is effective in the treatment of skin problems, anxiety and others. The oil is known for its antiseptic and soothing properties. When used after surgery, it provides relief from post-operative pain.

Ingredients:

- Jojoba oil (5 ml)
- Lavender oil (3 drops)

Directions:

Mix the carrier oil and the essential oil in a dark colored glass bottle and shake well.

To Use:

Apply topically over the affected areas twice a day.

You can also mix the essential oil in water for application. Tea tree oil and Helichrysum oil are also effective in treating eczema.

Carrot seed oil is multipurpose oil that has skin healing and rejuvenating properties. This essential oil can effectively treat numerous skin problems like psoriasis, eczema and others.

Ingredients:

- Rosehip seed oil (5 ml)
- Carrot Seed Oil (3 drops)

Directions:

Mix rosehip seed oil (carrier oil) and carrot seed oil (essential oil) in a glass container. Shake the container well, rolling it between your hands and turning the bottle upside down to mix the oils well.

To Use:

Clean the affected area and apply the mixture twice a day.

Helichrysum oil is also effective in treating

psoriasis and other skin ailments.

Blackheads

Blackheads are every woman's bane but men suffer from them too. They usually occur on the chin, cheeks or the nose and just turn into a zit at the most inopportune moment without any consideration for the circumstances or event. No, blackheads definitely are not the things to have on your face. Helichrysum essential oil is effective for the treatment of all skin ailments, including blackheads.

Ingredients:

- Sunflower oil (1/2 ounce)
- Apricot oil (1/2 ounce)
- Helichrysum (6 to 8 drops)

Directions:

Mix the carrier oils, i.e. sunflower and apricot oil, in a glass container and shake well. Add six to eight drops of helichrysum essential oil to this carrier oil mix and shake well again so that the oils are mixed well.

To Use:

Take a few drops of the oil and massage on your skin in gentle circular motions. Alternately, you can saturate a cotton ball with a few drops of the oil and apply over the blackheads. Use it once a day.

In addition to helichrysum essential oil, lavender oil, Neroli essential oil, Roman chamomile oil, clary sage oil, mandarin essential oil, Sandalwood essential oil, tea tree essential oil, carrot seed oil and frankincense oil are also effective in treating blackheads. Mix any of these oils individually with the carrier oils and apply on the blackheads.

Treatment of Acne

Every person goes through the acne stage. Acne does not necessarily appear during the teenage years. It can also make an impromptu appearance during the adult stages of life (known as adult acne). Tea tree oil is an effective essential oil that helps treat acne. It is an important ingredient in many acne treating creams and lotions.

Ingredients:

- Jojoba oil (0.6 ounce)
- Grape seed oil (0.4 ounce)
- Tea tree oil (7 drops)

Direction:

Mix jojoba oil and grape seed oil in 60/40 ratio, i.e. sixty percent of jojoba oil and forty percent of grape seed oil. The mixture should be one ounce in weight. Mix it in a glass bottle and shake it well. To this mixture, add six to seven drops of tea tree essential oil. Mix it well again, shaking the bottle in an up and down motion.

To Use:

Clean your face and apply a few drops of this oil mixture to the affected areas twice a day.

Other essential oils such as helichrysum, clary sage, lavender, frankincense, mandarin and sandalwood are also effective in the treatment of acne.

Treatment of Oily skin

Tea tree essential oil is derived from tea tree that is found in Australia. It is a natural antiseptic, which also helps in treating oily skin by dissolving excess sebum and eliminating acne causing bacteria.

Ingredients:

- Tea Tree Oil (1 drop)

Direction:

Just dab one drop of tea tree essential oil on cotton ball and apply over your face. Do this once a day.

In addition to tea tree essential oil, eucalyptus oil, chamomile, mandarin, orange, cypress, lavender, bergamot and Ylang Ylang also effectively treat oily skin.

Treatment of Body Odor

Rosemary essential oil belongs to the mint family. The essential oil is derived from the Rosemary plant, which is popularly used in cooking. The essential oil helps in curbing body odor by restricting the growth of bacteria that causes odor.

Ingredients:

- Beeswax (2 ounces)
- Rosemary essential oil (7 to 8 drops)

Directions:

Melt the beeswax in a pot over low heat. When the beeswax melts, add the rosemary essential oil and mix well. Let the mixture cool.

To Use:

Take a small amount of the mixture under your arms everyday to eliminate body odor.

You can also add lemongrass, or lavender essential oils for fragrance.

Treatment for Brittle Nails

The aroma of grapefruit essential oil is citrusy and fresh. It is uplifting and energizing. Grapefruit essential oil contains d-limonene, a powerful antioxidant that nourishes nails and skin.

Ingredients:

- Flaxseed oil (3 tablespoons)
- Grapefruit essential oil (15 drops)

Directions:

Mix the flaxseed oil with grapefruit essential oil in a glass bottle. Look for pure essential oil for maximum benefit. Shake the mixture well.

To Use:

Rub a few drops of the mixture on your nails twice a day.

You can also use other citrus essential oils such as lemon, sweet orange or lime.

Treatment for Dandruff

Tea tree essential oil is one the most popular oils used to treat dandruff and other scalp problems. It has anti-inflammatory and anti-fungal properties and is also used in many hair products meant for dandruff treatment.

Ingredients:

- Regular shampoo (8 ounces)
- Tea tree essential oil (10 drops)

Directions:

Mix 10 drops of tea tree essential oil to 8 ounces of your regular shampoo. Mix the shampoo well with the essential oil.

To Use:

 Apply shampoo to wet hair and let the tea tree essential oil shampoo remain in your hair for 5 minutes. Rinse off the shampoo with cool water.

You can also use rosemary essential oil, and

hempseed essential oil for treating dandruff.

Scar and Stretch Mark Reduction

Chamomile essential oil is one of the most powerful essential oils that are used in aromatherapy. This oil has anti-inflammatory properties and cools down the body. It helps in the reduction of scars and stretch marks.

Ingredients:

- Bath water
- Chamomile essential oil (10 drops)

Directions:

Add 10 drops of chamomile essential oil to your bath water and let it sit for a while.

To Use:

Take bath with the essential oil infused bath water for reduction in scars and stretch marks.

Lavender essential oil is also high effective in the treatment of stretch marks.

Treatment of Wrinkles

Rose essential oil is very effective in preventing and reducing wrinkles. The essential oil is extracted from cabbage roses and mixed with carrier oils such as almond, hazelnut or jojoba oils and applied on skin.

Ingredients:

- Jojoba oil (2 tablespoons)
- Rose essential oil (15 drops)

Directions:

Mix 2 tablespoons of jojoba oil and 15 drops of rose essential oil in a clean glass bottle. Shake the bottle well to mix the oils.

To Use:

Cleanse your face and steam it. When you face is still damp, massage a few drops of the oil. This helps in penetration of the oil and reduces wrinkles. Leave it on the face as the oil is easily absorbed into skin.

You can also use lavender oil, rosemary, geranium or Neroli instead of rose essential oil as the former is much more easily available.

Dry Skin

Lavender essential oil is refreshing and soothing. This versatile oil is used for the treatment of many skin, scalp and body problems, including dry skin. You can either make a scrub for your dry skin using the oil or just add 7 drops of lavender essential oil to your bath water for best results.

Ingredients:

- Lavender oil (6 drops)
- Peppermint oil (2 drops)
- Elder flowers/chamomile (1 tablespoon)
- Cornmeal (1 tablespoon)
- Oatmeal (2 tablespoons)

Directions:

Mix the dry ingredients and grind them to a fine powder. Add the peppermint and lavender essential oils to the powder and mix well. Store in an airtight container.

To Use:

Cleanse your face. Add just enough of the above mixture to a teaspoon of water and apply on damp face. Let it remain for a couple of minutes and then scrub your face gently. Rinse with water. Use it every day instead of face wash or soap.

Treatment of Arthritis

Peppermint essential oil is highly effective in the treatment of joint pains and arthritis. The anti-inflammatory and anesthetic oil helps alleviate joint pains.

Ingredients:

- Grape seed Oil (3.5 ounces)
- Peppermint Oil (60 drops)

Directions:

Mix the two oils together in a glass bowl and shake well.

To Use:

Apply the mixture to the affected areas topically and massage gently. Use it twice a day for pain relief.

Treatment of Abdominal Cramping or Pain

Clary sage essential oil has estrogen like properties that help relieve abdominal cramping and pain.

Ingredients:

- Almond oil (1 teaspoon)
- Clary sage oil (1 drop)
- Rose oil (1 drop)
- Lavender Oil (2 drops)

Directions:

Mix the oils in a clean glass bottle, shaking it well to mix the oils.

To Use:

Massage a few drops of the oil on your abdomen for relief from abdominal cramps and pain.

Treatment of Acid Reflux

Lemon essential oil contains a substance called d-limonene that helps in treating acid reflux. The essential oil is for consumption and, therefore, you must ensure that you use only CPTG essential oils.

Ingredients:

- Water (16 ounces)
- Lemon oil (2 drops)

Directions:

Mix the oil in the water and stir it well.

To Use:

Drink the water throughout the day for relief from acid reflux. Lemon oil eliminates acid from esophagus, throat lining and stomach.

Treatment Cold and Flu

There are numerous essential oils for treatment of cold and flu. These oils such as eucalyptus, rosemary, lavender, frankincense and Myrtle are used in combination for their balancing and anti-histamine effect.

Ingredients:

- Lavender (7 drops)
- Myrtle (5 drops)
- Frankincense (6 drops)
- Eucalyptus (2 drops)
- Rosemary (1 drop)
- Dill (2 drops)

Directions for Use:

Mix the oils together and massage on the soles of your feet, hands and over chest.

You can also diffuse the oils for relief.

Geranium essential oil is extracted from geranium flowers. It contains soothing and calming properties that make it ideal for the treatment of depression and sadness.

Ingredients:

- Bergamot oil (6 drops)
- Geranium oil (3 drops)
- Jojoba oil (2 ounces)

Directions:

Mix the oils in a glass bottle and shake well.

To Use:

You can either massage the oil on your body or add it to your bath water. Soak in the water for at least 20 minutes. If you leave out the jojoba oil, you can also make an air spray.

Lavender essential oil is also effective in treating depression and sadness.

Treatment of Fever

Essential oils such as lavender and peppermint are beneficial for treatment of fever. They have anti-inflammation properties and soothe the body.

Ingredients:

- Evening Primrose oil (15 ml)
- Eucalyptus oil (2 drops)
- Lavender oil (2 drops)
- Peppermint oil (2drops)
- Black pepper and tea tree oil (1 drop each)
- Rosemary oil (1 drop)

Directions:

Mix the oils together in a glass bottle and shake well.

To Use:

Take a few drops of the oil and massage the back of your neck, temples, feet and hand soles.

Treatment of Inflammation

Helichrysum oil is one of the best essential oils containing anti-inflammatory properties. It helps reduce all kinds of inflammations.

Ingredients:

- Jojoba oil (1 ounce)
- Helichrysum oil (8 drops)

Directions:

Mix the two oils in a plastic or glass bottle and store in a cool and dark place.

To Use:

Massage the oil on affected areas.

Stress Relief

Lavender oil is used in body lotions, bath salts and massage oils because it reduces pulse rates and eliminates stress.

Ingredients:

- Jojoba oil (1 ounce)
- Lavender oil (8 drops)

Directions:

Mix the lavender essential oil to Jojoba carrier oil and shake well.

To Use:

Use it as a diffuser or spray in your room. It is a stress buster and very effective.

Treatment of Fatigue

Carrot seed oil has excellent rejuvenating properties. Therefore, it is used in combating fatigue.

Ingredients:

- A bowl of water
- Carrot seed oil (3 drops)

Directions:

Add the oil in a bowl of hot water and stir it.

To Use:

Bend over the bowl and cover your head and face with a thick towel. Inhale the steam.

Treatment of Anxiety

Lavender essential oil is one of the most versatile essential oils used in aromatherapy. It is used in the treatment of stress and anxiety.

Ingredients:

- Lavender Essential oil (2 drops)
- Frankincense (2 drops)

Directions:

Mix the two oils together and diffuse in your room. Alternatively, you can also massage the oils on your hand and feet soles.

Oils such as wild orange, lemon, bergamot and patchouli are also excellent for reducing anxiety.

Headaches

Three essential oils are used for treatment of headache – Lavender oil, Roman chamomile and clary sage. They have soothing and anti-inflammatory properties.

Ingredients:

- Bath water
- Lavender oil (6 drops)

Directions:

Add the oil to warm bath water.

To Use:

Soak in the bath water for 20 minutes.

You can also use clary sage or roman chamomile instead of lavender for similar results.

Treatment of Insect Bites and Stings

Many people are allergic to insect bites and stings. They may need medical help. However, essential oils such as peppermint oil provide instant relief.

Ingredients:

- Jojoba oil (1 ounce)
- Peppermint oil (6 drops)

Directions:

Mix the oils in a plastic bottle.

To Use:

Clean the bitten area with warm water and apply a drop of the blend on the bite.

Lavender oil prevents inflammation and muscle spasms. It relieves tension and reduces back pain.

Ingredients:

- Sweet almond oil (1 ounce)
- Lavender oil (8 drops)

Directions:

Mix the oils in a bottle and store in a cool and dark place.

Other oils such as frankincense, clary sage, yarrow and chamomile also have inflammatory properties and soothe the pain away.

To Use:

Massage a few drops of the oil on your back for relief from back pain.

Treatment of Hormonal Transitions (Menopause and PMS)

Hormonal problems can be treated with essential oils such as chamomile, marjoram, lavender and Melissa. You can inhale these oils or massage them on your abdomen. If the oils are fit for consumption, then you can make herbal tea for relief.

Ingredients:

- Lavender, Chamomile, Clary sage, Marjoram, Geranium and ginger oils (12 drops combined)
- Jojoba oil (1 ounce)

Directions:

Mix the oils in a glass bottle and shake well.

To Use:

Massage a few drops on the abdomen, lower back and hips for cramps relief.

Pain Relief

Wintergreen essential oil is the most effective oil for relief from pain. It contains methyl salicylate that can provide immediate pain relief.

Ingredients:

- Wintergreen essential oil (4 drops)
- Jojoba oil (1 ounce)

Directions:

Mix the oils in a glass or plastic bottle and shake well before application.

To Use:

Massage 3 drops on the painful area or diffuse in the room.

Respiratory Conditions

Chamomile and peppermint essential oils are effective in providing relief from respiratory problems. They are anti-inflammatory and have soothing properties.

Ingredients:

- German chamomile (4 drops)
- Frankincense (2 drops)
- Jojoba oil (1 ounce)

Directions:

Mix the carrier and essential oils in a plastic or glass bottle and shake them well.

To Use:

Apply on the chest and cover immediately with flannel.

This mixture is also very helpful in case of asthma attack. For respiratory problems of nose, eucalyptus, tea tree and peppermint oil are effective; for chest congestion, mix lavender, hyssop, rosemary and eucalyptus oil and massage over chest.

Essential oils are fast becoming a popular alternative to modern medicine. They are effective and have no side effects. In addition to providing relief from physical ailments, they also promote emotional well-being.

Final Words

I hope you must have not only enjoyed this book but also tried few recipes. If you want to let others know about your experience, please post your valuable and constructive reviews. Your feedback matters and it really does make a difference.

I would greatly appreciate your comment because your review is going to help me improve and update my work. If you found any error or anything you suggest to change or add in this, do let me know at satenyada@yahoo.in and I promise a quick personal response.

Your review is going to make a true experience for other readers and help them make their buying decision easier. If you'd like to leave a review then all you need to do is go to review section of book and click on "Write a customer review".

Again, thanks for your time, trust and support. Also by ADISH Books are the following books –

Essential Oils Beauty Secrets: Make Beauty Products at Home for Skin Care, Hair Care, Lip Care, Nail Care and Body Massage for Glowing, Radiant Skin and Shiny Hairs

Lemon: 50 Plus Recipes for Skin Care, Hair Care, Home and Laundry Cleaning along with Lemonade, Vegan, Curd, Chicken, Cookies, Cakes and Desserts

Scrubs and Masks: 50 Simple Natural Homemade Recipes for Glowing Radiant and Younger Skin by Exfoliation, Moisturizing and Nourishing Facial Masks for All Skin Types

The Amazing Coconut Oil Miracles : Simple Homemade Recipes for Skin Care, Hair Care, Healthy Smoothies, Muffins, Soup, Salad, Chicken and Desserts Along With Weight Loss and Detoxification Plan

Juicing Magic: 50+ Recipes for Detoxification, Weight Loss, Healthy Smooth Skin, Diabetes, Gain Energy and De-Stress

www.ingramcontent.com/pod-product-compliance
Lightning Source LLC
Chambersburg PA
CBHW070303290526
45791CB00003B/1065